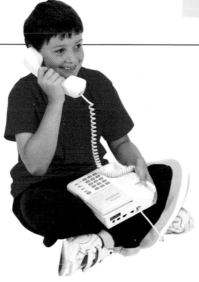

# When it's hard to
# hear

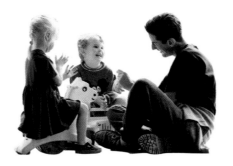

## Judith Condon

**W**
**FRANKLIN WATTS**
LONDON • SYDNEY

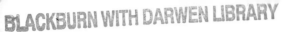
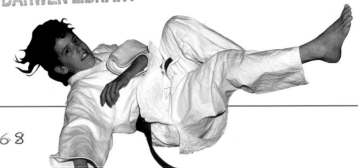

First published in 1998 by Franklin Watts,
96 Leonard Street,
London EC2A 4XD

Franklin Watts Australia,
56 O'Riordan Street,
Alexandria, Sydney, NSW 2015

This book was created and produced for
Franklin Watts by
**LN Books**,
B2, Ivinghoe Business Centre,
Blackburn Road,
Houghton Regis,
Bedfordshire LU5 5BQ

Project management: Ruth Nason
Design: Carole Binding
Illustration: Jane Cradock-Watson
Photography: Peter Silver
Consultants: Deborah Jones-Stevens,
Heathlands School, St. Albans; Beverley
Matthias/REACH Resource Centre; Dr
Philip Sawney; William Sawney

Printed and bound in Belgium

ISBN 0 7496 4531 8 (pbk)

Dewey Decimal Classification 617.8

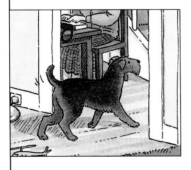

**Can you find where the Hearing Dog appears in this book?**

**Acknowledgements**
The author would like to thank all the
people featured in this book: in particular,
Maria Sampson, Alex Fergus, Leonidas
Constantinides and family, Sarla Meisuria
and members of the Asian Deaf Women's
Association, James Strachan, and Shelly
Begum. Also for their help and advice:
Philippa Rose, Jo Campbell, Jenny Bourke,
Mr and Mrs Warren, Karen Sampson,
Nishma Shah and Xiu Mei Tian-Clarke.

The photographs on pages 4t, 12, 14, 15, 21t
and 23bl were taken by Peter Silver. Thanks
are also expressed to the following for their
permission to reproduce photographs: BBC
Subtitling, p 13b; BT Corporate Picture
Library, pp 7r, 22b, 23t, c, r; BDA, p 16t;
Eye Ubiquitous (Bennett
Dean), pp 4br, 26b;
Format (Paula
Solloway), pp 6, 20t;
Mike Gerrard, p 17bl,
21b; Hearing Dogs for
Deaf People, p 17r;
Heathlands School,
p 20b; Peter J. Millard:
cover l, tr; NDCS, p 16t;
Retna (Michael Putland),
pp 11, 27; Science Photo
Library (James King-Holmes),
pp 10, 11t; Colin Sims
Photography, p 16b;
Tony Stone
Images (James
Strachan),
p 22t; James
Strachan, p 22c;
The Guardian
(Garry Weaser),
p 13t; The Times
(Adrian Brooks),
cover br, p 17tl;
Topham
Picturepoint,
p 26t; TRIP
(S. Grant), p 7l.

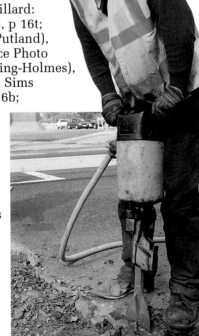

# Contents

Introduction                          6

Think about sounds                    8

Types of deafness                    10

Meet some people who are deaf        12

The Deaf Community                   16

At home                              18

Everybody's learning!                20

At work                              22

Out and about                        24

Famous people                        26

Glossary                             28

Useful information                   29

Index                                30

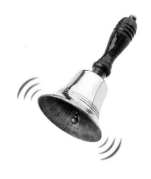

# Introduction

In this book you will meet several people who are deaf. If they were not in this book, you might not specially notice them, out and about, at work and school, playing and having fun.

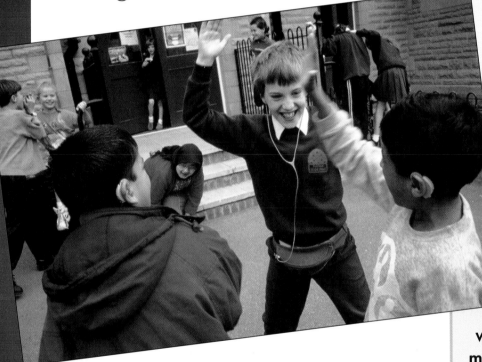

Some wear hearing aids, which make sounds louder for them.

## Lip-reading

To help work out what you are saying, some deaf people use the skill of lip-reading. They also notice your body language.

**Listen!**
**What does 'listening' mean? How is it different from hearing?**

**When the teacher says 'Listen!', it doesn't just mean 'Stop talking!'**

**On the right is how Chinese people write 'listen'. This Chinese writing helps us see what listening is all about.**

**The Chinese word is made up of shapes which represent: ear, you, eyes and heart.**

**So, listening means more than hearing. It means using your eyes and your feelings, as well as your ears. It means giving someone else your time and your patience.**

**Deaf people may not be able to use their hearing as much as other people. But they can certainly be excellent listeners.**

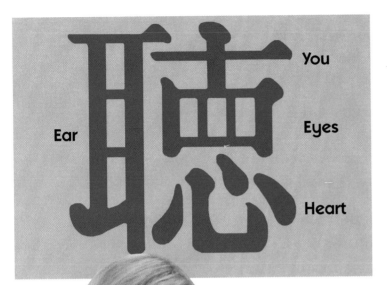

Ear  You  Eyes  Heart

◀ The Chinese characters which make up the verb 'to listen'.

## Talking and listening

Talking and listening are skills we don't often stop to think about. But what is it like when it's hard to hear? And what if you can't hear anything at all?

If you can't hear, how do you learn words, or what they mean? Can you understand what your teacher is saying? Can you enjoy watching television and videos?

How can you tell when the phone is ringing, and communicate with your friend on the other end of the line?

The people in this book have answers to these questions, and to many more.

## Sign language

Some deaf people use a special language, called sign language. Their arms, hands and face do the 'talking' and their eyes do the 'listening'.

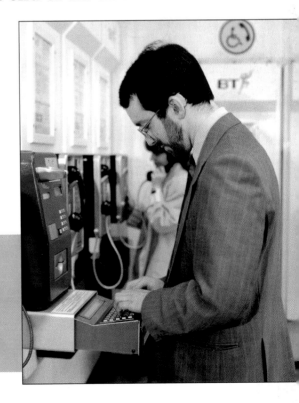

▶ Many deaf people use text phones. This is a text pay-phone at a railway station.

# Think about sounds

How many sounds can you find in these pictures?

Try grouping the sounds you find under different headings, such as 'Human sounds', 'Animal sounds', 'Warning sounds', 'Entertaining sounds'...

Sometimes it is hard to hear what someone is saying because there is so much noise going on all around. That kind of noise is called background noise. Can you find examples of background noise in these pictures?

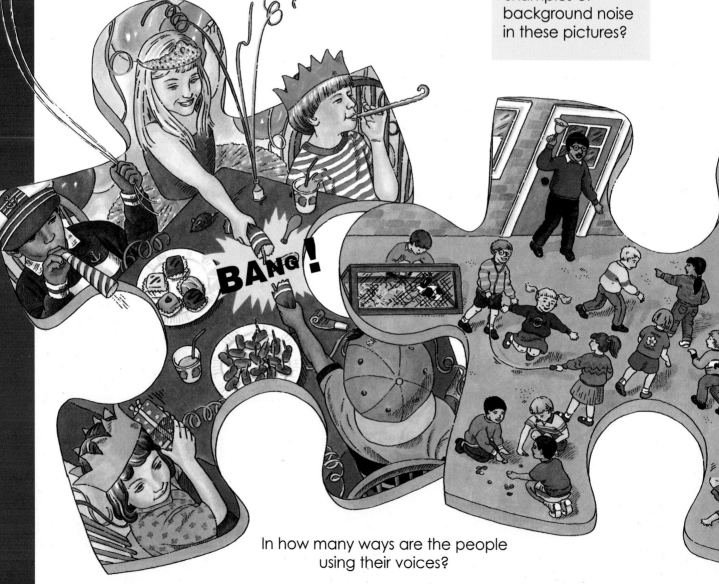

BANG!

In how many ways are the people using their voices?

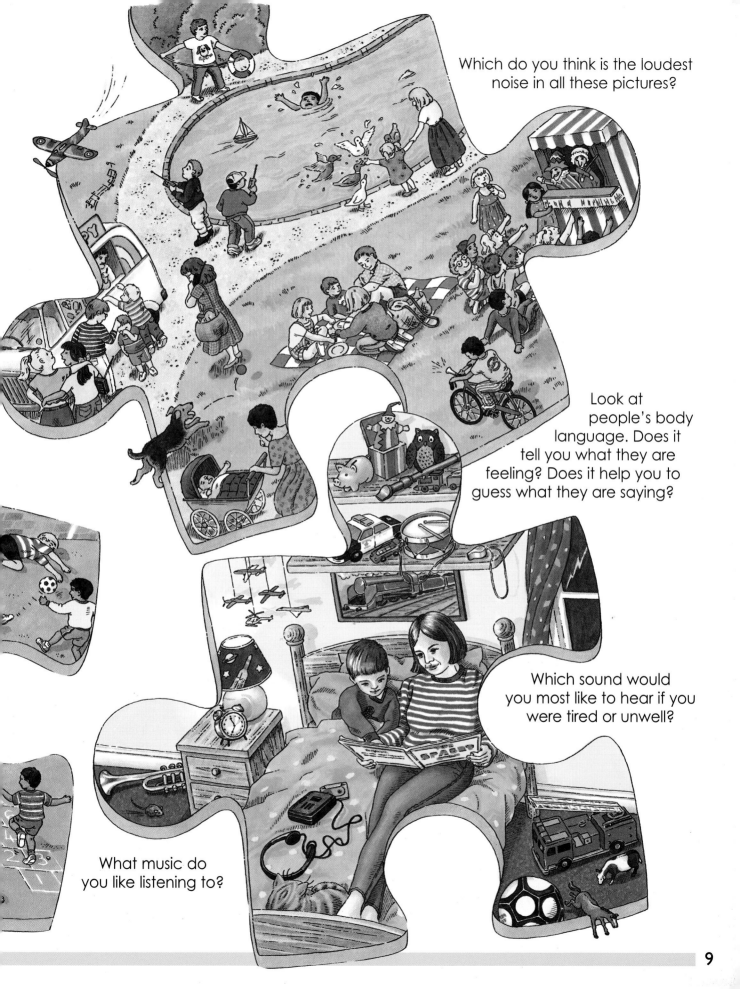

Which do you think is the loudest noise in all these pictures?

Look at people's body language. Does it tell you what they are feeling? Does it help you to guess what they are saying?

Which sound would you most like to hear if you were tired or unwell?

What music do you like listening to?

# Types of deafness

Did you know that dogs hear sounds that are too faint or too high for humans to hear? Perhaps dogs think all humans are a bit deaf!

## Levels of deafness

Deaf is a general word. But not all deafness is the same.

Tests can measure a person's level of deafness. It may be mild, moderate, severe or profound.

▼ Even small babies can have their hearing tested.

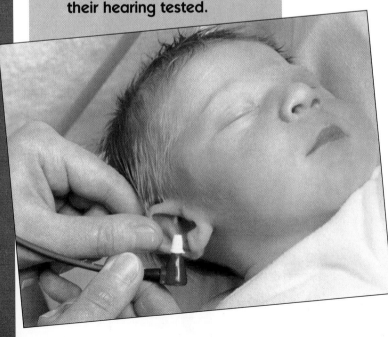

## Lip-reading

Most deaf people use lip-reading to help them understand speech. It is not easy!

Look in the mirror and say 'Poor, More, Bore'.

All three words look the same! Still, many deaf people are experts at lip-reading.

If YOU talk to someone who lip-reads, be sure to face them, and don't speak too fast.

## Causes of deafness

About one in a thousand babies in Britain is born deaf.

Sometimes deafness may be passed on to a baby by its parents' genes. This can happen even if neither parent is deaf. Sometimes a baby is made deaf because the mother is ill as the baby forms inside her.

Other people become deaf later in their life. The cause may be an illness or an accident.

## Learning to talk

Think of how you learned to talk, by copying other people. Learning to talk is hard for people who are deaf, and hardest of all for people who were born deaf.

▼ The 'visual ear' computer turns sounds into shapes, to help the person learn to say words.

## Glue ear

Some children have 'glue ear'. Fluid inside the ear does not drain away, and this makes it hard to hear. Glue ear tends to clear up as you grow. Then your hearing gets better too.

### Tinnitus
Someone with tinnitus has a buzzing or ringing in the ears that goes on all the time. It does not come from outside, but from inside. It can be tiring and upsetting.

## Loud noise

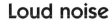

A rock group called The Who played louder than any other group in the 1960s. Their guitarist Pete Townsend (below) became deaf.

Being close to loud noise – music, machinery, or explosions – can cause permanent damage to the ears.

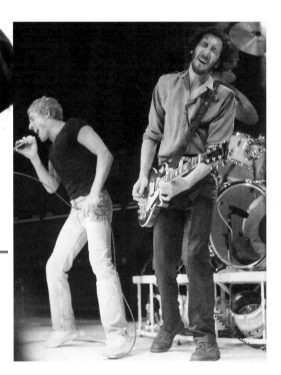

## Elderly people

Our hearing tends to weaken as we grow old. Low sounds may be easier to hear than high ones. Sometimes one ear works better than the other.

Have you ever been asked to talk on someone's 'good side'?

# Meet some people who are deaf

## Maria's story

My name is Maria Sampson and I am 11. This is me with my cat Tigger. He's a tabby. I have a sister and a brother, but Tigger likes me best!

I go to Hazelwood Junior School. I'm the only deaf person in my class. I have loads of friends.

Things I like include writing stories about animals, and doing judo – as you can see. Recently I won my Green Belt.

I keep a diary so I don't forget things. Recently I went on a school journey to the Isle of Wight. It was hot. We did canoeing and swimming.

Next year I am going to secondary school. I already have a friend there. I'm looking forward to it.

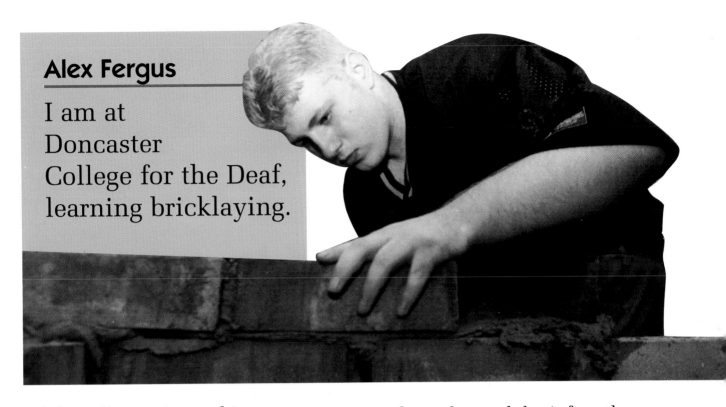

## Alex Fergus

I am at Doncaster College for the Deaf, learning bricklaying.

I did work experience this year and, by coincidence, the man who was my boss has a deaf daughter. He spoke slowly and clearly so I could understand.

I was surprised when he said I should train to be a manager. He made me confident in many ways.

You see, there are not many deaf people, so friendship is important to us. I like to go out with my friends and communicate in sign language. It's quick and simple.

Technology helps a lot. I like to watch TV. Usually, the actors speak too fast and don't face the front. It's difficult to understand them. But subtitles change that.

Speaking to someone on the telephone is incredibly difficult, because you can't see the lips. I phone my friends a lot on the minicom (a kind of text phone). You type what you are saying and the other person types back.

In my spare time I love reading.

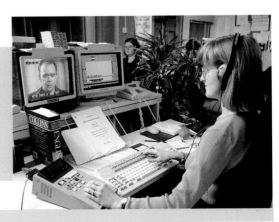

▶ Subtitles are words at the bottom of the TV picture. This is the unit at the BBC where subtitles are added to TV programmes.

## Sarla starts a special club

Sarla Meisuria was born in India, but came to Britain as a baby. She went first to a school for deaf children, then to a mainstream (ordinary) school.

Sarla in her office, using a text phone. She wears a plain colour rather than a patterned fabric. This makes it easier for other people to see when she uses sign language.

She says: 'As well as English, I know Hindi and some Gujarati, British Sign Language, and a bit of Asian Sign.'

When she grew up, Sarla realized that Asian deaf women needed their own club.

### Hearing aids

Some hearing aids are worn behind the ear, and have a tube taking sound into a fitted ear piece. Some fit completely into the ear.

A hearing aid doesn't give its wearer perfect hearing, but it can be very helpful. It amplifies (increases the loudness of) sounds. It works best where there is no background noise.

A hearing aid contains a tiny microphone and amplifier, and is run by a battery.

Most hearing aids have a volume control and a special 'T' setting, to connect with a loop system (see page 18).

Nearly 2 million people in Britain wear hearing aids in one or both ears.

Sarla explains: 'Many people do not understand what deafness means. Deaf women from Asian families can be very isolated.'

Sarla and her husband have three children. None of them is deaf. Even with her family to look after, in 1992 she found time to put her plan into action.

'I did not know anything about running a group. I learned the hard way!'

Now the Asian Deaf Women's Association has its own office, with three deaf workers and two volunteers. Lots of support and training are offered to the women who come along.

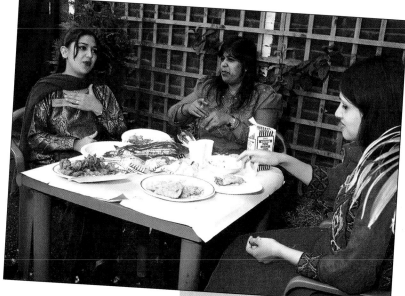

▲

The Asian Deaf Women's Association is in east London. This photo shows some of the women enjoying a chat over lunch.

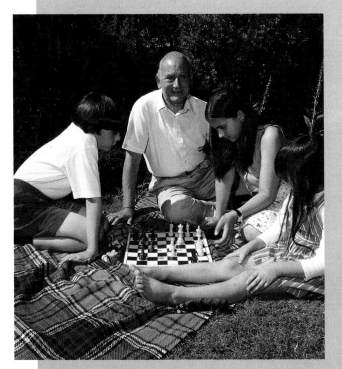

## Leonidas Constantinides

Leonidas is teaching three of his grandchildren to play chess.

He came from Cyprus to London, where he worked as a compositor – making up pages of type ready for printing.

Since he retired, he does not hear as well as he used to. It helps if people speak clearly, and if there is no background noise.

# The Deaf Community

Deaf people enjoy getting together. They share interests and experiences. They meet up through clubs and magazines.

**BSL (British Sign Language) is used by about 50,000 deaf people, their families, and those who work with them.**

**It is not a copy of English, but a quite separate language with its own rules – and jokes!**

▶ **Magazines produced by the British Deaf Association and the National Deaf Children's Society.**

British Deaf news
AUGUST 1997  BDA Members £1.00  Non-Members £1.2
The magazine for Deaf people
Deaf people
BRITISH DEAF ASSOCIATION

Contents
2 Opinions
3 News
4 Behind the News
5 Feature:
CACDP - 3

Row contin

TALK
ISSUE NO: 164  Summer 1997
The Magazine of The National Deaf Children's Society
FREE GUIDE TO DISABILITY LIVING ALLOWANCE

## Sign language

Of all the things deaf people share, the most important is sign language.

Sign is the special language of the Deaf Community. It uses movements of the arms, hands and face instead of spoken sounds. It is very expressive. The movements are fluid and fast.

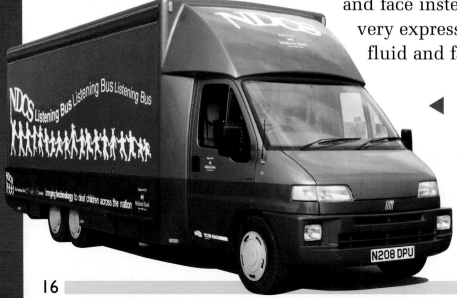

◀ **The 'Listening Bus' of the National Deaf Children's Society travels round the UK, taking the latest toys and equipment to show to deaf children and their parents.**

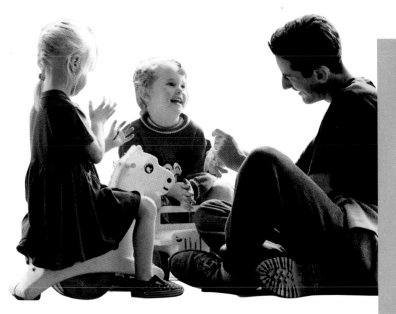

## Learning sign language

What was the first language you learned? Probably you learned it at a very young age, long before you learned to read. We need a language, to think and communicate with.

Many children who are born deaf learn sign language as their first language. Later, they learn English or whatever language is spoken around them.

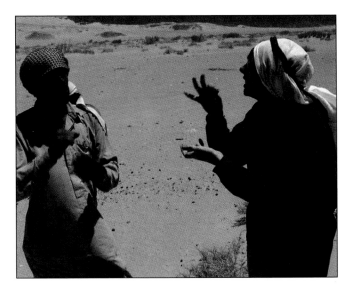

## Hearing Dogs

Some deaf people have a specially trained Hearing Dog.

When the dog hears a sound – for example, the telephone or the microwave 'pinging' – he touches his owner, and leads him or her to the right place.

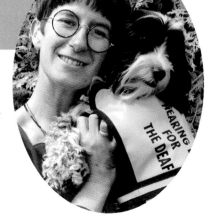

▶ **Actress Charlotte Moulton-Thomas and her Hearing Dog, Ouzo.**

## Around the world

There are many different sign languages around the world.

In Sinai, Egypt, 8 per cent of the Bedouin people are born deaf or become deaf as children. Most Bedouin learn to sign, and so no-one feels left out.

Bedouin sign is not the same as BSL. But British visitors to Sinai, using BSL, manage to communicate with the Bedouin – as Christine (on the right of the photo) found out!

# At home

In this house the artist has included many things that are useful for people who are deaf. How many can you spot?

A peripatetic (travelling) teacher has come to visit the little girl, who is deaf. The Hearing Dog already knows that she has arrived!

 Vibrating pad connected to the alarm clock

 Transmitter, sending radio signals to pager

 Loop amplifier

 Computer, linked to the Internet

 Smoke alarm flashes as well as making a sound

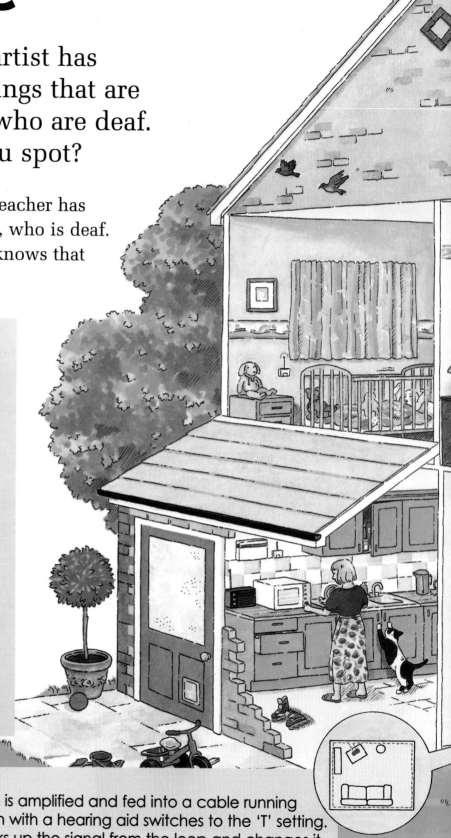

**Loop system**
Sound from the television is amplified and fed into a cable running round the room. A person with a hearing aid switches to the 'T' setting. The hearing aid then picks up the signal from the loop and changes it back into sound. Since the TV set does not have to be turned up loud for the deaf person to hear, others in the room are happy too.

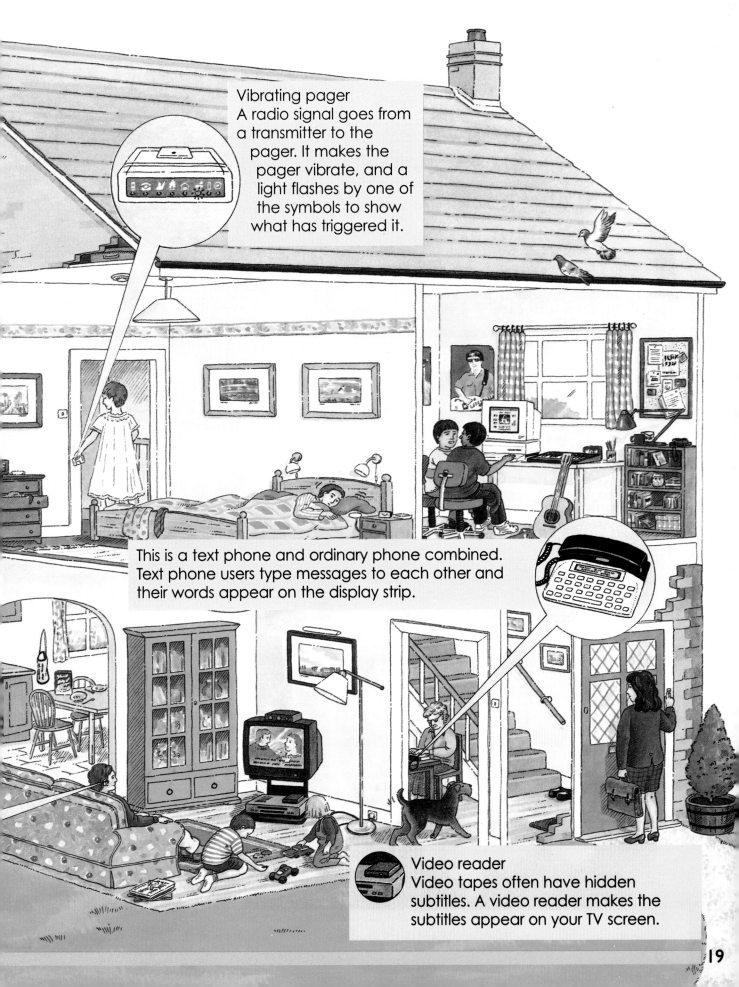

**Vibrating pager**
A radio signal goes from a transmitter to the pager. It makes the pager vibrate, and a light flashes by one of the symbols to show what has triggered it.

This is a text phone and ordinary phone combined. Text phone users type messages to each other and their words appear on the display strip.

**Video reader**
Video tapes often have hidden subtitles. A video reader makes the subtitles appear on your TV screen.

# Everybody's learning!

About 60,000 deaf children are at school in Britain.

Most go to mainstream (ordinary) schools. A smaller number go to special schools for deaf children. Here the teachers use sign language as well as English. The children may also have lessons with speech therapists.

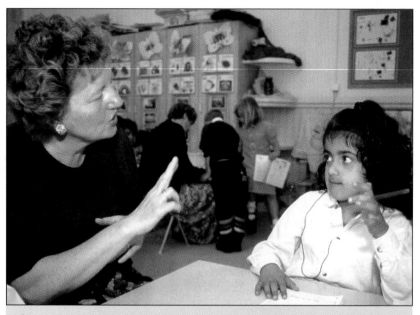

▲ At mainstream schools, deaf children are taught with all the other children. But they may also have individual help from a specially trained teacher of the deaf.

▼ A classroom specially designed for deaf pupils.

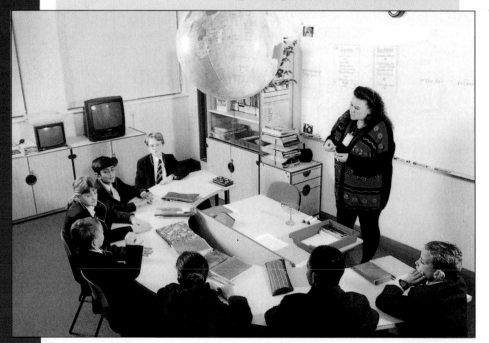

## Special equipment

In special schools, classrooms are sound-treated, to minimise background noise.

The teacher wears a transmitter and the pupils have radio aids.

Tables in a horse-shoe shape allow everyone to see the face of whoever is talking.

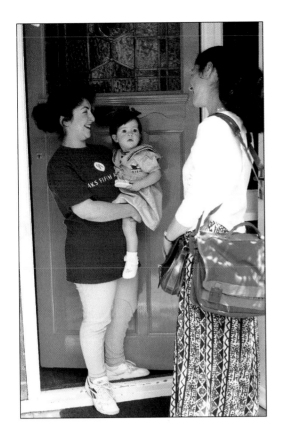

## Early learning

Philippa Rose is a peripatetic teacher, specially trained to teach deaf children.

Here she is visiting baby Nicole Warren and her mother. Nicole is the only deaf member of the family. Philippa uses sign language so that Nicole will begin to learn it.

Now Nicole's parents, grandparents and aunties are going to sign language lessons. They want to be able to communicate with Nicole too!

▼ A BSL interpreter translates into sign language what the tour guide is telling this group of people on an educational holiday.

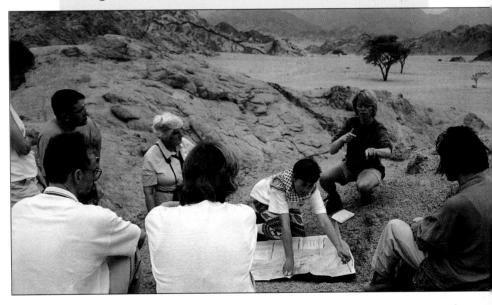

## Access

Many organizations try to *include* people with disabilities. This policy is sometimes called 'access'.

For people who are deaf, this may mean providing a sign language interpreter.

In the past, people with disabilities were often *excluded*. They tended to miss out on opportunities such as further education.

New technology has helped. So has a change in other people's attitudes. Increasingly it is recognized that people who are deaf should have equal opportunities to gain the best out of life.

# At work

Some deaf people work in the Deaf Community; some in the hearing community.

Text phones, fax machines and video phones are particularly useful. With a video phone you can see the person on the other end of the line.

People who are deaf can also communicate with hearing people, anywhere in the world, using 'Typetalk'.

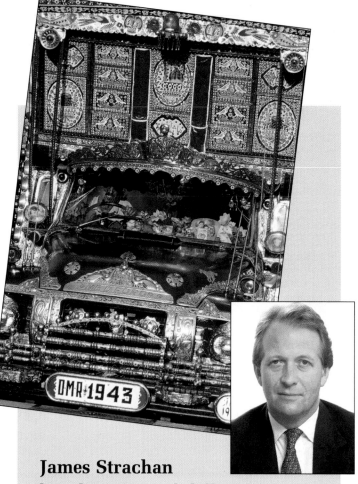

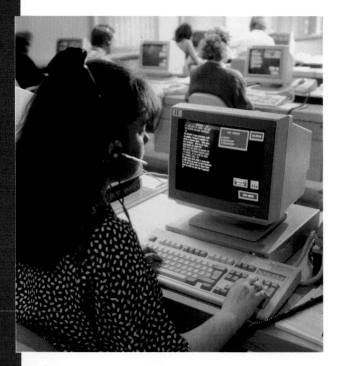

▲ A Typetalk operator. (See page 23.)

**James Strachan** has done several different kinds of work, including being a travel photographer.

His photographs for books and magazines are of far-away places and unusual subjects – like this decorated lorry in Pakistan!

James is profoundly deaf.

Before becoming a photographer, he was managing director of a big international bank. Now he is head of the Royal National Institute for Deaf People.

## Go ahead! How to use Typetalk

Here's how to telephone someone who uses a text phone. But get permission first!

- Ring the Typetalk number – 0800 515152 – using an ordinary telephone.

- A Typetalk operator (like the one on page 22) answers and asks the number you want to call.

- She dials this number and, using her text phone, makes contact with the person.

- She asks you what you want to say and types this in.

- The other person reads your message on the screen of his text phone, and types his reply.

- The operator reads these words on her text phone screen and speaks them to you.

- When you hear the words 'Go ahead', it's your turn to speak again.

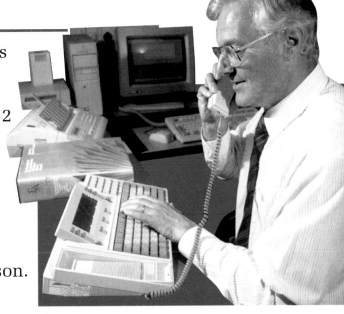

▲ Receiving a Typetalk call.

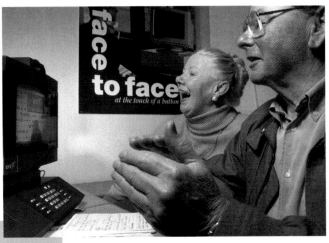

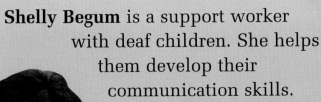

**Shelly Begum** is a support worker with deaf children. She helps them develop their communication skills.

Shelly came to Britain from Bangladesh when she was nine. Like her family, she spoke Bengali, so she had to learn English and British Sign Language too.

▲ The parents of Paul Hebblethwaite, in London, used the video phone to speak to Paul when he was in New Zealand.

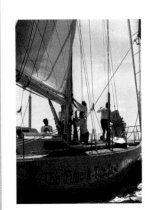

Paul, who is profoundly deaf, was taking part in a round-the-world yacht race.

# Out and about

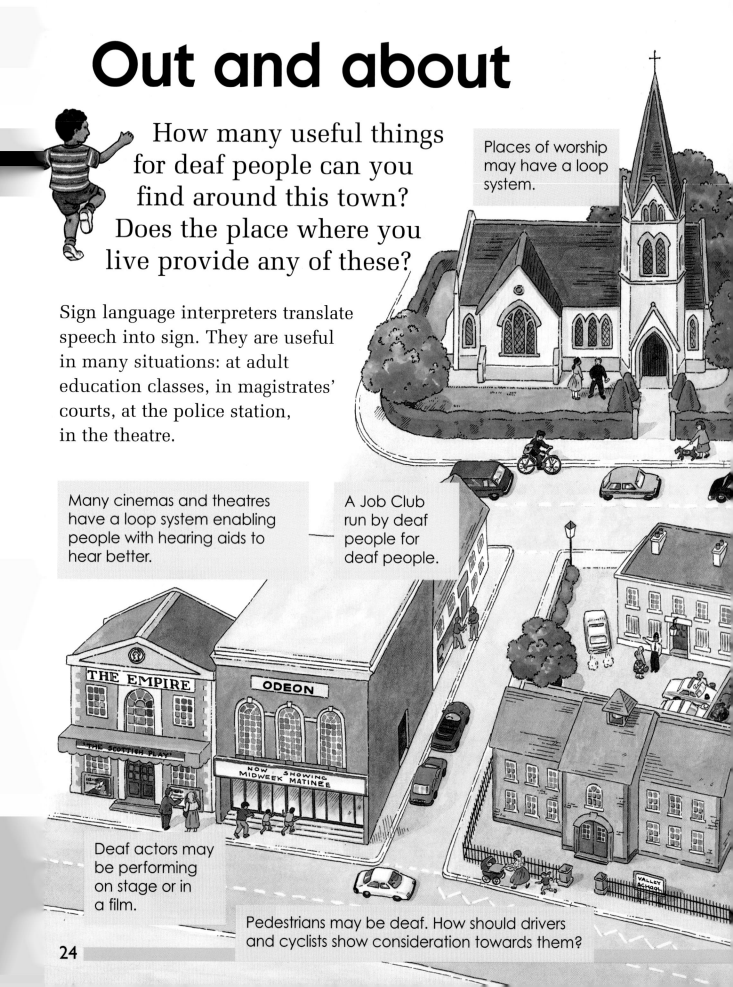

How many useful things for deaf people can you find around this town? Does the place where you live provide any of these?

Sign language interpreters translate speech into sign. They are useful in many situations: at adult education classes, in magistrates' courts, at the police station, in the theatre.

Places of worship may have a loop system.

Many cinemas and theatres have a loop system enabling people with hearing aids to hear better.

A Job Club run by deaf people for deaf people.

Deaf actors may be performing on stage or in a film.

Pedestrians may be deaf. How should drivers and cyclists show consideration towards them?

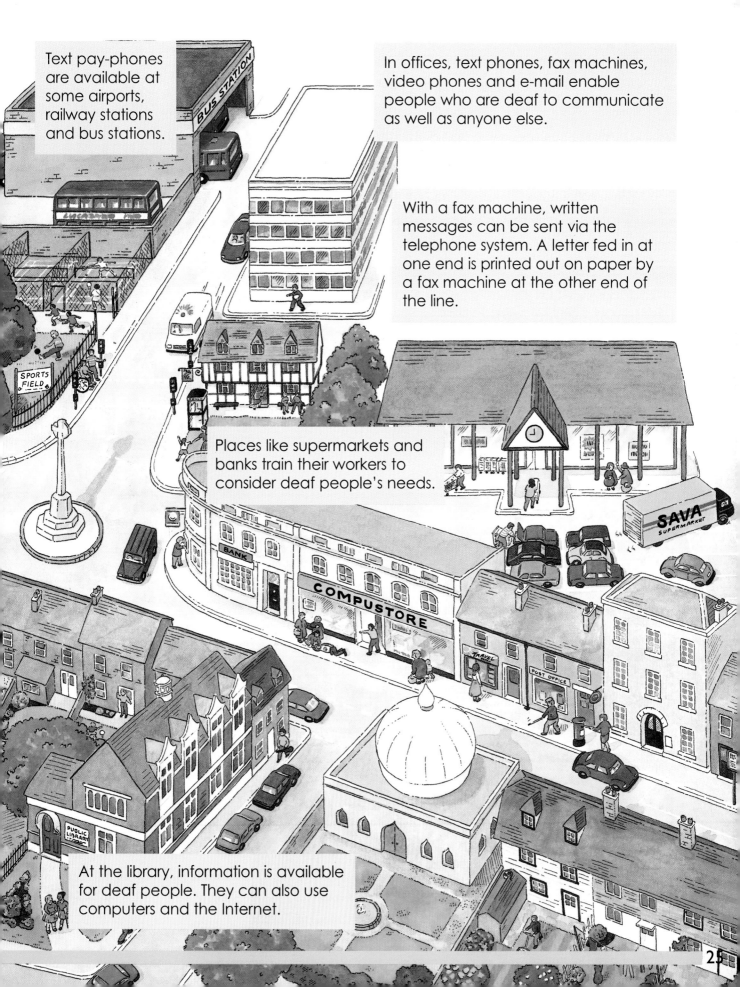

Text pay-phones are available at some airports, railway stations and bus stations.

In offices, text phones, fax machines, video phones and e-mail enable people who are deaf to communicate as well as anyone else.

With a fax machine, written messages can be sent via the telephone system. A letter fed in at one end is printed out on paper by a fax machine at the other end of the line.

Places like supermarkets and banks train their workers to consider deaf people's needs.

At the library, information is available for deaf people. They can also use computers and the Internet.

# Famous people

## Beethoven

Born in Germany in 1770, Ludwig van Beethoven is one of the best-loved composers of all time. He went gradually deaf in his late twenties, but still continued to write great and dramatic music, which has inspired people worldwide. Part of his Ninth Symphony is used as the anthem for the European Union.

## David Bower

David (right) is a deaf actor who graduated from Reading University's course in Theatre Arts, Education and Deaf Studies. He played Hugh Grant's brother in the hugely popular film *Four Weddings and a Funeral*.

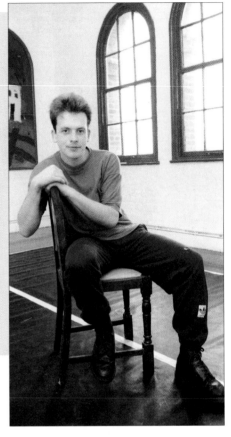

One hundred years ago, riveters working in ships' boilers often went deaf. They worked in a small space and their work was very noisy. This form of deafness became known as boiler-makers' disease.

Nowadays there is a law to protect people at work. Anyone exposed to loud or explosive noise must be given ear protectors. What jobs can you think of where people wear ear protectors?

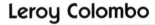

## Leroy Colombo

Leroy was a profoundly deaf long-distance swimmer and life-saver who lived in Texas. Between 1920 and 1960 he saved 907 lives, some of them from boats on fire. He is recorded in the *Guinness Book of Records* as the World's Greatest Life Saver.

## Evelyn Glennie

Evelyn Glennie, who is profoundly deaf, is a world-famous musician. She senses the vibration of the music, and uses that sense when playing percussion instruments such as the xylophone.

## Goya

Francisco de Goya was a Spanish painter, born in 1746. At age forty-six he suffered an illness that left him temporarily paralysed, and deaf for the rest of his life. His experience of human suffering led him to paint imaginative and sometimes terrifying paintings.

## Emma Nicholson

As a Member of Parliament in the 1990s, Emma became an expert lip-reader. Many people did not realize that she was moderately deaf. Sometimes she would lip-read what her opponents were whispering to each other on the other side of the House of Commons, and use it to her advantage.

## Kenny Walker

Black American football player Kenny Walker went deaf when he was two. He played for the University of Nebraska, and then for the top-flight club, the Denver Broncos – only the second deaf player to become a professional. But he suffered discrimination (unfair treatment) at the club and later won a case against it. His story is told in a film called *Silent Cheers*.

## Michelangelo

This great Italian artist and sculptor (1475-1564) suffered from tinnitus. We do not know for sure what caused the terrible buzzing in his ears. But he spent years hammering noisily at blocks of marble, to make wonderful statues. Though tinnitus often made him depressed, he worked until he died, aged eighty-eight.

# Glossary

**body language**
This 'language' consists of the way a person sits or stands, the movements he or she makes, and the expressions on his or her face. All these things give information about what the person is thinking, feeling and saying.

**BSL**
British Sign Language.

**cochlear implant**
Some deaf people have an operation during which an electronic device (a kind of 'receiver') is placed inside their ear. Afterwards they also wear a box outside the ear, which works like a transmitter, sending sound signals to the receiver.

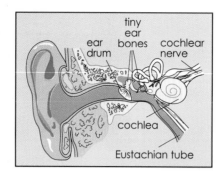

This creates a tiny electric current in a nerve leading to the brain. The device, called a cochlear implant, gives the person a limited level of hearing.

**genes**
biological units which pass on characteristics, such as eye colour, from parents to their children.

**glue ear**
Fluid in the middle ear should drain away down the Eustachian tube. But sometimes it gathers behind the eardrum, causing infection and loss of hearing. Doctors sometimes prescribe anti-biotics, or insert small drainage tubes called grommets.

**profound deafness**
Many experts say that the term 'profoundly deaf' should only be used to describe people born with no hearing, or very little hearing, or who became deaf before they learned to talk.

**speech therapist**
a person trained to help children and adults who have difficulty speaking, or speaking clearly.

Sign language has existed for hundreds of years. But a conference in 1880 decided that spoken language was better than sign. Signing was banned from schools in many countries, and children were even punished for using it!

Teachers believed signing would make children lazy about trying to hear and speak. Fortunately, deaf people kept signing alive and in the 1970s ideas changed. Now people can use whichever language suits them best.

# Useful information

A mail-order catalogue of British Deaf Association material is available from:
**Big D Company Ltd,**
P O Box 20,
Coleford,
Gloucester GL16 8YP
The catalogue includes posters to introduce hearing children to sign, and video-tapes of children's stories in BSL.

For older children and adults, it lists books on deaf history and culture; videos including *A Beginner's Guide to Sign*; and a BDA information pack covering deaf culture, working with deaf people, etc.

A school pack is available from:
**Hearing Dogs for Deaf People,**
Training Centre,
London Road (A40),
Lewknor,
Oxon OX9 5RY
tel 01844 353 898 (voice and text)
fax 01844 353 099

For information on **Typetalk** call Freephone 0800 800 848.

## Organizations in Australia

**Deafness Resource of Australia,**
33Argyle Street,
Parrammatta NSW 2150
tel 02 9204 2970

**Deaf Education Network,**
Exeter Road,
Homebush NSW 2140
tel 02 9764 4600

## Organizations in the UK

**British Deaf Association (BDA),**
1-3 Worship Street,
London EC2A 2AB
tel 0171 588 3520
minicom 0171 588 3529 (text)
fax 0171 588 3529

**National Deaf Children's Society (NDCS),**
15 Dufferin Street,
London EC1Y 8PD
tel 0171 250 0123 (voice and text)
fax 0171 251 5020

**Royal National Institute for Deaf People (RNID),**
19-23 Featherstone Street,
London EC1Y 8SL
tel 0171 296 8000
minicom 0171 296 8001
fax 0171 296 8199

**REACH** (National Research Centre for Children with Reading Difficulties),
Wellington House,
Wellington Road,
Wokingham, Berkshire RG40 2AG
tel 0118 989 1101 (voice and minicom)
fax 0118 979 0989
(Works to meet reading needs of children who are deaf.)

**Shops, banks, offices and other organizations display this symbol to show that they consider the needs of people who are deaf.**

# Index

access **21**
alarms **18, 19**
Asian Deaf Women's
  Association **14, 15**

babies **10**
background noise **8, 14,**
  **15, 20**
BDA (British Deaf
  Association) **16**
Bedouin **17**
Beethoven **26**
Begum, Shelly **23**
body language **6, 9**
boiler-makers' disease
  **26**
Bower, David **26**
BSL (British Sign
  Language) **16, 17, 23**

cinemas **24**
clubs **14, 15, 16, 24**
cochlear implant **28**
Colombo, Leroy **26**
computers **11, 19, 25**
Constantinides, Leonidas
  **15**

Deaf Community **16**
deafness, causes **10, 11**
deafness, levels of **10**
dogs **10, 17, 18, 19**

ear protectors **26**

elderly people **11**
equal opportunities **21**

fax machine **22, 25**
Fergus, Alex **13**

genes **10**
Glennie, Evelyn **27**
glue ear **11, 28**
Goya **27**

hearing aids **6, 14, 18,**
  **24**
Hearing Dogs **17, 18,**
  **19**
hearing test **10**
Hebblethwaite, Paul **23**

interpreters **21, 24**

lip-reading **6, 10, 27**
listening **6, 7**
Listening Bus **16**
loop system **14, 18, 24**

magazines **16**
Meisuria, Sarla **14, 15**
Michelangelo **27**
minicom **13**

NDCS (National Deaf
  Children's Society) **16**
Nicholson, Emma **27**
noise **11, 26**

pager **18, 19**
police station **24**

radio aids **20**
Rose, Philippa **21**

Sampson, Maria **12**
schools **12, 14, 20, 21,**
  **28**
shops **25, 29**
sign language **7, 13, 14,**
  **16, 17, 20, 21, 23, 28**
Sinai **17**
Strachan, James **22**
subtitles **13, 19**

talking **7, 11, 13**
teachers **18, 20, 21, 28**
telephones **7, 13, 14, 17,**
  **19, 22, 23, 25**
television **13, 18, 19**
theatres **24**
tinnitus **11, 27**
Townsend, Pete **11**
Typetalk **22, 23**

video **19**
video phone **22, 23**

Walker, Kenny **27**
Warren, Nicole **21**
Who, The **11**
work **13, 14, 15, 22, 23,**
  **24, 25, 26**